CHRONIC PAIN SOLUTIONS

Integrative Therapies For Lasting Relief

Discover A Comprehensive Guide To Managing Chronic Pain Through A Combination Of Conventional And Alternative Therapies

DR. BRIDGET PROMISE

CHAPTER ONE

Introduction

Chronic pain is a complicated and widespread health problem that affects millions of people worldwide. Chronic pain, as opposed to acute pain, which is often a warning sign of injury or sickness and dissipates over time, lasts for long periods, frequently months or even years.

This persistent pain may have a substantial influence on many elements of a person's life, including physical, mental, and social problems. In this investigation, we will look at the nature of chronic pain, its influence on everyday living, and the efficacy of established pain management techniques.

Understanding chronic pain:

Chronic pain is distinguished by its persistence, which extends much beyond the normal recovery period associated with a particular injury or sickness.

It may be caused by a variety of illnesses such as arthritis, nerve injury, or musculoskeletal issues. Unlike acute pain, which often serves a protective purpose, chronic pain frequently develops into a disorder in its own right, requiring specialist care.

Chronic pain is caused by a variety of complicated causes. Persistent pain signals may be delivered to the brain long after the primary injury has healed. This condition, known as maladaptive plasticity, includes alterations in the neural system that maintain pain sensations.

Furthermore, psychological elements such as stress, worry, and depression may worsen the experience of chronic pain, resulting in a feedback loop between the physical and mental components of suffering.

The special effects of Chronic Pain on our Daily Life:

The consequences of chronic pain go well beyond the physical experience of anguish. Individuals suffering from chronic pain often notice a significant impact on their everyday lives.

Physical constraints may impair mobility and the capacity to accomplish normal tasks, lowering one's overall quality of life. Simple actions like walking, standing, or sitting for long periods may become difficult problems.

Chronic pain also has a profound emotional impact. Constant discomfort may cause increased stress, worry, and depression.

The inability to participate in previously loved activities or maintain social contacts might exacerbate feelings of loneliness and dissatisfaction. Sleep difficulties are especially prevalent in those with chronic pain, increasing the total effect on mental health.

Individuals with chronic pain may struggle to engage in social activities or meet household and career commitments, causing social dynamics to shift. This may lead to feelings of estrangement and a progressive deterioration of the support networks required to cope with chronic pain. As a result, the holistic effect of chronic pain goes beyond physical suffering, permeating the emotional and social worlds and influencing a person's total well-being.

Traditional approaches to pain management:

Historically, pain treatment techniques have concentrated on symptom relief rather than addressing the root causes of persistent pain. Traditional methods often include the use of medicines, physical therapy, and, in some situations, surgical procedures. Nonsteroidal anti-inflammatory medications (NSAIDs) and opioids are routinely used to treat pain by reducing inflammation or altering pain perception.

Physical therapy is another common technique that includes exercises and treatments to enhance strength, flexibility, and mobility.

While these approaches may be helpful for some people, they often fail to address the multifaceted nature of chronic pain.

Medications may cause dependence or unwanted side effects, while physical therapy may not necessarily result in long-term gains.

CHAPTER TWO

Limitations of Conventional Treatments:

Despite the extensive use of conventional pain treatment methods, their limits have become more evident. Medications, especially opioids, involve the danger of addiction and may only give short-term comfort without treating the underlying cause of persistent pain.

Furthermore, the risks associated with long-term pharmaceutical usage often exceed the benefits.

Physical therapy, although useful to some, may not be universally successful since its effectiveness is frequently dependent on the nature of the chronic pain and individual reactivity. Surgical operations are designated for specialized instances, and they carry their own set of risks and problems.

Furthermore, conventional methods often overlook the psychological and emotional components of chronic pain. Mental health therapies such as cognitive-behavioral therapy, mindfulness, and stress management are increasingly acknowledged as critical components of total pain management. Ignoring these aspects may jeopardize the overall effectiveness of therapy and the individual's capacity to live with and manage chronic pain effectively.

Chronic pain is a complex and complicated health condition that goes beyond physical discomfort. Understanding its intricacies, recognizing its influence on everyday life, and critically examining established methods of pain treatment are all necessary steps toward delivering more complete and effective solutions. As we continue to investigate novel strategies that take into account the holistic aspect of chronic pain, there is a promise for better results, a higher quality of life, and a more compassionate approach to assisting patients on their road to pain alleviation and well-being.

Exploring Integrative Therapies: A Comprehensive Approach to Pain Management

Pain, whether acute or chronic, has a substantial influence on an individual's quality of life. Traditional medical treatments often concentrate on treating symptoms rather than addressing the root causes. In recent years, there has been an increased interest in integrative treatments that take a holistic approach to pain management. These treatments acknowledge the interconnection of the mind and body, stressing the significance of treating the whole person. In this inquiry, we will look at integrative treatments, especially the mind-body connection, holistic methods, dietary tactics, and exercise as crucial components in chronic pain alleviation.

Mind-Body Connection in Pain Management

The mind and body are inextricably linked, and their effect

on one another is clear. Integrative treatments use the mind-body link to provide holistic pain management. Mindfulness meditation, guided imagery, and biofeedback are techniques that use the mind's capacity to modify pain perception.

Mindfulness meditation, based on ancient techniques, entails increasing awareness of the present moment without judgment. Regular mindfulness practice has been demonstrated in studies to lessen symptoms linked with chronic pain disorders while also enhancing a feeling of well-being and general mental health.

Guided imagery is another effective technique in the integrative toolset. Individuals may use visualization methods to shift their attention away from pain, boosting relaxation and mental clarity. This may be especially effective for persons enduring stress-related or psychosomatic discomfort.

Biofeedback adopts a more scientific approach by giving users real-time information regarding physiological processes, such as heart rate or muscular tension. Individuals may learn to regulate their body's reaction to pain by exercising conscious control over these processes, resulting in better pain management.

Holistic Approaches to Chronic Pain Relief

Integrative treatments adopt a comprehensive approach to pain management, acknowledging that the physical, emotional, and spiritual elements of a person are intertwined. Acupuncture, chiropractic treatment, and massage therapy are all holistic techniques.

Acupuncture, derived from ancient Chinese medicine, involves the insertion of tiny needles into particular spots on the body. This ancient technique seeks to regulate the flow of energy or "qi" throughout the body. Numerous studies show that acupuncture may be useful in lowering pain and increasing general well-being, making it a significant component of integrative pain care.

Chiropractic therapy focuses on the interaction of the spine and the neurological system. By treating misalignments in the spine, chiropractors strive to decrease pain and increase the body's capacity to recover itself. Chiropractic adjustments have been proven to be especially useful for ailments such as lower back pain and headaches.

Massage treatment, with its origins in diverse cultural traditions, includes the manipulation of soft tissues to induce relaxation and reduce muscular tension. Beyond its physical advantages, massage treatment may have a good influence on emotional well-being, adding to a holistic approach to pain alleviation.

CHAPTER THREE

Nutritional Strategies for Alleviating Pain

Diet has an important part in general health, and specific dietary techniques may be used to control and relieve chronic pain. Anti-inflammatory diets high in fruits, vegetables, and omega-3 fatty acids have gained popularity due to their ability to alleviate pain caused by illnesses such as arthritis and inflammatory disorders.

Turmeric, a spice rich in the anti-inflammatory chemical curcumin, has shown promise in relieving pain and increasing function in people with osteoarthritis and rheumatoid arthritis. Including turmeric in one's diet or taking pills may provide a natural solution to pain treatment.

Omega-3 fatty acids, found in fatty fish such as salmon and mackerel, are anti-inflammatory. According to studies, increasing omega-3 consumption may help those with joint discomfort or inflammatory disorders.

Maintaining a healthy weight is also essential for treating chronic pain. Excess weight may worsen osteoarthritis and cause physical discomfort. A balanced and healthy diet, along with regular exercise, may help with weight control and reduce discomfort.

Exercise and Physical Therapy for Long-Term Relief:

Physical exercise is an essential component of integrative pain treatment, supporting both physical and emotional well-being. Exercise and physical therapy not only improve flexibility and strength, but they also produce endorphins, the body's natural pain relievers.

Walking, swimming, and cycling are all low-impact workouts that might be very useful to those suffering from chronic pain. These exercises assist in preserving joint function and limit the likelihood of additional damage. Additionally, water exercise offers buoyancy, which reduces joint impact while still providing a cardiovascular workout.

Physical therapy, under the supervision of skilled specialists, seeks to enhance mobility and functioning via specific exercises and treatments. Stretching, strengthening exercises, and manual therapy may all treat the underlying causes of pain and provide long-term relief.

Finally, investigating integrative treatments for pain management provides a comprehensive and diversified approach to treating chronic pain. Individuals may empower themselves to manage pain more successfully by acknowledging the deep relationship between the mind and body, combining holistic approaches, using anti-inflammatory food choices, and engaging in regular exercise.

As integrative medicine advances, the prospect for enhanced pain treatment and general well-being becomes more promising.

Alternative therapies include acupuncture and massage.

Alternative treatments in pain management have received widespread attention for their ability to supplement established medical approaches. Acupuncture and massage are two popular treatments in this field, each providing distinct approaches to pain relief and general well-being.

Acupuncture, which originated in ancient Chinese medicine, is the insertion of tiny needles into particular spots on the body. These spots connect to energy routes, and stimulation is said to enhance the flow of energy, or "qi," which restores balance and reduces pain. Acupuncture has shown promise in treating a variety of pain disorders, including osteoarthritis, migraines, and back pain.

Massage treatment, on the other hand, is the manipulation of soft tissues to improve circulation, relieve muscular tension, and induce relaxation. Massage's tactile nature not only relieves physical discomfort but also improves mental health. Regular massage treatments help many people recover from illnesses such as muscular tightness, tension headaches, and fibromyalgia.

According to research, both acupuncture and massage may cause the release of endorphins, the body's natural painkillers, offering pain relief as well as an improvement in mood. Furthermore, these treatments provide a comprehensive approach to pain, taking into account both the physical and emotional elements.

Mindfulness and meditation for pain reduction.

Mindfulness and meditation have emerged as effective pain-reduction techniques. Mindfulness is the cultivation of an awareness of the present moment without judgment, while meditation includes a variety of activities aimed at gaining mental clarity and tranquillity.

These strategies enable people to have a different connection with their pain, promoting acceptance and decreasing emotional responses that might increase suffering. Mindfulness-Based Stress Reduction (MBSR) programs, which involve mindfulness meditation, have been demonstrated to be effective in treating chronic pain.

Participants often report improved pain intensity, functional restrictions, and psychological well-being.

Mindfulness practices allow people to shift their attention away from painful feelings, giving them a sense of control over their experiences. Individuals who acquire a nonjudgmental awareness may be able to interrupt the loop of stress and anxiety-induced pain amplification. Furthermore, mindfulness and meditation help calm the neurological system, improving pain perception and tolerance.

CHAPTER FOUR

Innovative Technologies for Pain Management

Technological advancements have opened up new horizons in pain treatment, providing creative methods that seek to improve both accuracy and efficacy. One example is the use of virtual reality (VR) and augmented reality (AR) in pain distraction treatment.

These technologies distract attention away from pain stimuli by immersing people in virtual settings or overlaying digital aspects of the actual world, delivering a distinct kind of analgesia.

Virtual reality settings, for example, may transfer people to relaxing landscapes or engaging activities, providing a sensory-rich experience that competes with pain signals. This not only acts as a diversion, but it also allows the brain to analyze several inputs at the same time, lowering pain perception.

Another significant technical innovation is the introduction of neurostimulation devices. These technologies, such as transcutaneous electrical nerve stimulation (TENS) units, send moderate electrical impulses via nerve pathways, interrupting pain signals and increasing endorphin production. Implantable technologies, such as spinal cord stimulators, provide more focused treatment for chronic pain problems, resulting in long-term alleviation.

The Role of Supportive Therapies: Counselling and Psychotherapy

Supportive treatments, such as counseling and psychotherapy, are essential for pain management because they address the psychological and emotional aspects of the experience. Chronic pain frequently hurts mental health, resulting in illnesses such as depression, anxiety, and stress. Integrating psychological therapy into a complete pain management strategy helps improve general well-being and coping skills.

Counseling offers a secure area for people to communicate their pain-related ideas and feelings. Cognitive-behavioral therapy (CBT), a popular technique, assists clients in identifying and changing negative thinking patterns and behaviors connected with pain. This may result in a more adaptive reaction to pain.

Psychotherapy looks further into the emotional components of pain, examining how prior events and relationships influence an individual's sense of pain. Individuals may increase resilience, enhance emotional control, and promote a feeling of empowerment in pain management by using a variety of therapeutic strategies.

The use of counseling and psychotherapy in pain treatment recognizes the link between physical and emotional well-being. Individuals who treat the emotional components of pain may see a more thorough and long-term improvement in their overall quality of life.

Complimentary Herbal and Supplemental Approaches

In their search for holistic pain management, many people look toward alternative herbal and supplementary techniques to enhance traditional treatments. Herbs and nutritional supplements have been used throughout civilizations for ages, with proponents suggesting possible anti-inflammatory, analgesic, and relaxation-inducing effects.

Popular herbal medicines include turmeric for its anti-inflammatory benefits and valerian root for its relaxing characteristics. These botanical choices often come in a variety of formats, such as teas, capsules, and topical applications. Individuals should check with healthcare specialists before adopting herbal therapies, as interactions with drugs and possible adverse effects must be considered.

Dietary supplements may also help with pain management, with compounds such as omega-3 fatty acids, glucosamine, and chondroitin sulfate being studied for possible joint health advantages. While some studies show favorable results, the efficacy of these supplements varies by person, and contact with healthcare practitioners is essential to assure safety and appropriateness.

To summarize, the combination of alternative treatments, mindfulness and meditation, new technology, supporting therapies, and complementary herbal and supplementary techniques provides a diverse and tailored approach to pain relief. Individuals may improve their well-being and quality of life by identifying and dealing with the physical, emotional, and psychological elements of pain.

Living with chronic pain may be a difficult and sometimes overwhelming experience that affects all aspects of one's life. While medicinal treatments are necessary, the importance of lifestyle changes in long-term pain alleviation cannot be emphasized. This holistic approach understands that pain management extends beyond typical medical treatments and focuses on individualized tactics adapted to each individual's specific requirements.

Lifestyle Changes for Long-term Pain Relief

Lifestyle changes are frequently the first step toward long-term pain treatment. These adjustments are intended to treat the physical, emotional, and psychological components of chronic pain. They include developing healthy habits, changing daily routines, and making decisions that promote general well-being.

Physical Exercise and Exercise: Contrary to popular belief, participating in adequate physical exercise is frequently an important part of treating chronic pain. Walking, swimming, and yoga are all examples of gentle workouts that may increase flexibility, muscular strength, and general function. Physical exercise causes the production of endorphins, the body's natural painkillers, which contribute to a more happy outlook.

Dietary modifications: Nutrition is very important for overall health and may have a big influence on pain levels. Anti-inflammatory diets that include fruits, vegetables, and omega-3 fatty acids may help to decrease inflammation and discomfort. It is important to work with a healthcare practitioner or a nutritionist to develop a customized dietary plan that is tailored to your specific health issues and demands.

Sleep hygiene: Quality sleep is critical to the body's capacity to recover and deal with discomfort. Establishing appropriate sleep hygiene habits, such as sticking to a regular sleep schedule, having a pleasant sleeping environment, and avoiding stimulants before bedtime, may all help to improve sleep quality.

Stress Management Techniques: Chronic pain often exacerbates stress, which may further heighten pain perception.

Stress management practices including meditation, deep breathing exercises, and mindfulness may help stop the pattern. These routines encourage relaxation, decrease physical tension, and boost general mental health.

CHAPTER FIVE

Personalized Pain Management Plans

Every person's experience with pain is unique, and so should their pain management strategy. Personalized therapies include the unique nature of the pain, the individual's medical history, lifestyle, and preferences. To maximize success, healthcare professionals and patients collaborate on the development of these programs.

Multidisciplinary Care Teams: Personalized pain treatment often requires a multidisciplinary approach, in which several healthcare specialists work together to address various elements of pain. This might involve physiotherapists, psychiatrists, pain experts, and dietitians collaborating to give holistic treatment.

Medication Management: While lifestyle changes are important, drugs may also be used to manage chronic pain. A tailored approach to medicine strikes the correct balance between relieving pain and reducing adverse effects. Regular communication between patients and healthcare professionals is vital for adjusting drugs depending on individual reactions and changing conditions.

Alternative treatments: Complementary and alternative treatments may be beneficial components of individualized pain management strategies. Acupuncture, chiropractic treatment, massage therapy, and biofeedback are all possible options. Integrating various treatments depending on individual preferences and reactions adds layers to the overall pain management strategy.

Case Studies: Successes in Integrative Pain Management

Real-life success stories demonstrate the efficacy of integrative pain treatment techniques. Case studies give insight into the many methods by which people have found healing and reclaimed control of their lives.

Jane's Journey to Pain Relief: Jane, a middle-aged fibromyalgia patient, began a tailored pain treatment regimen that included physical therapy, cognitive-behavioral therapy, and aquatic exercise. Jane reported a dramatic decrease in pain levels, increased sleep, and general well-being because of her constant efforts and the support of her healthcare team.

Mark's Holistic Healing: To cope with persistent back pain, Mark included mindfulness meditation and yoga in his daily regimen. This comprehensive approach not only lowered his dependency on pain drugs but also gave him techniques to handle stress and improve his mental resiliency.

Overcoming Challenges on the Path to Pain Relief

The journey to long-term pain alleviation is not without obstacles. Individuals may experience setbacks, greater discomfort, or times of irritation. These difficulties must be identified and addressed proactively.

Dealing with flare-ups: Despite the greatest efforts to control pain, flare-ups may occur. A contingency plan, including specific ways to handle rising pain levels, is essential. This might include temporary changes in physical activity, more rest, or changes to the pain management strategy in consultation with healthcare specialists.

Emotional Resilience: Chronic pain may hurt mental health.

Emotional assistance, whether provided via therapy, support groups, or contact with loved ones, is essential. Developing emotional resilience is recognizing and managing the emotional consequences of hardship while maintaining a positive attitude.

Empowering Yourself: Advocacy and Self-Care

Empowerment is a key topic on the path to long-term pain treatment. Advocacy entails actively engaging in one's care, being knowledgeable about treatment alternatives, and successfully communicating with healthcare practitioners. Self-care, on the other hand, refers to everyday behaviors that promote health and improve pain management.

Patient Advocacy: Empowered people actively participate in their healthcare journey. This involves learning more about their illness, asking questions, and participating in decision-making processes. Patient advocacy goes beyond the individual and includes a collective effort to raise awareness about chronic pain and push for better pain treatment solutions at the societal level.

Self-care Practices: Self-care is an essential component of long-term pain treatment. This includes establishing realistic objectives, prioritizing enjoyable hobbies, and accepting one's limitations. Setting limits, practicing proper sleep hygiene, and incorporating fun activities into everyday life all contribute to a comprehensive self-care strategy.

Conclusion

Long-term pain treatment is a comprehensive, continuing process. Lifestyle changes, tailored pain management programs, success stories, overcoming obstacles, and self-empowerment are all interwoven components of a complete approach to treating chronic pain. Recognizing the uniqueness of each person's experience and adjusting techniques appropriately leads to a more successful and long-term road to alleviation.

Ultimately, the route to long-term pain alleviation is a collective effort by people, healthcare providers, and the larger community to improve the quality of life for those suffering from chronic pain.